Sensei Self Development

Mental Health Chronicles Series

Overcoming Self-Doubt and Low Self-Esteem

Sensei Paul David

Copyright Page

Sensei Self Development -
Overcoming Self-Doubt and Low Self-Esteem,
by Sensei Paul David

Copyright © 2024

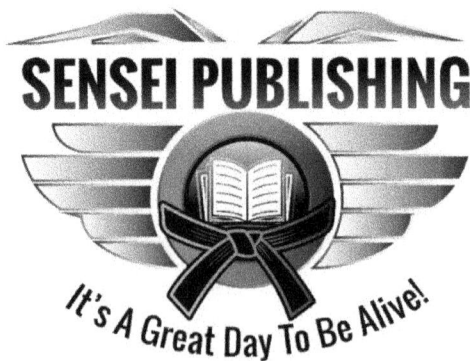

SENSEI PUBLISHING

It's A Great Day To Be Alive!

www.senseipublishing.com

@senseipublishing
#senseipublishing

Get/Share Your FREE SSD Mental Health Chronicles at

www.senseiselfdevelopment.care

or

CLICK HERE

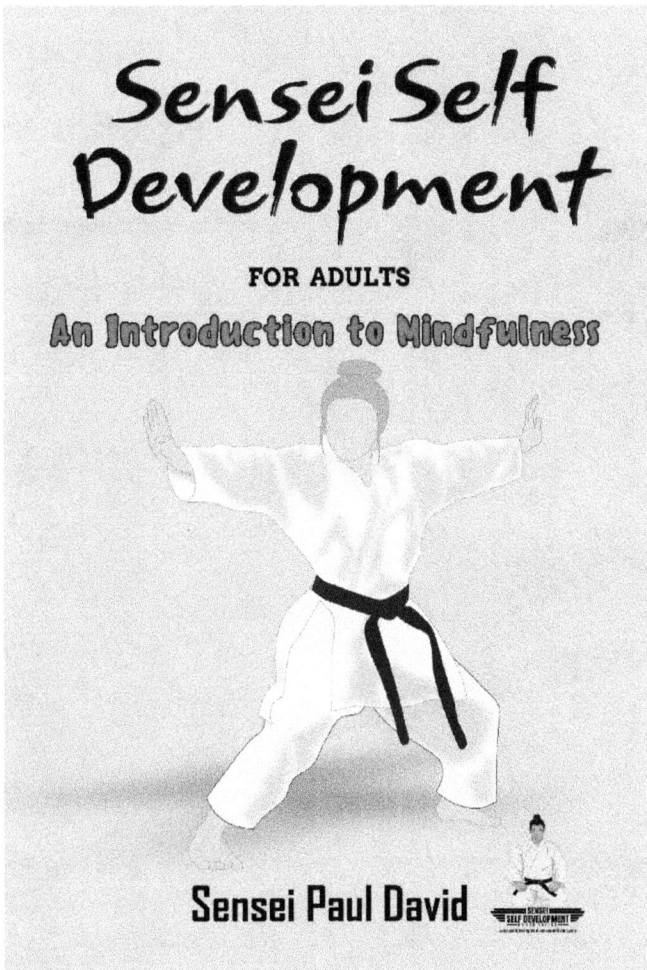

Check Out The SSD Chronicles Series CLICK HERE

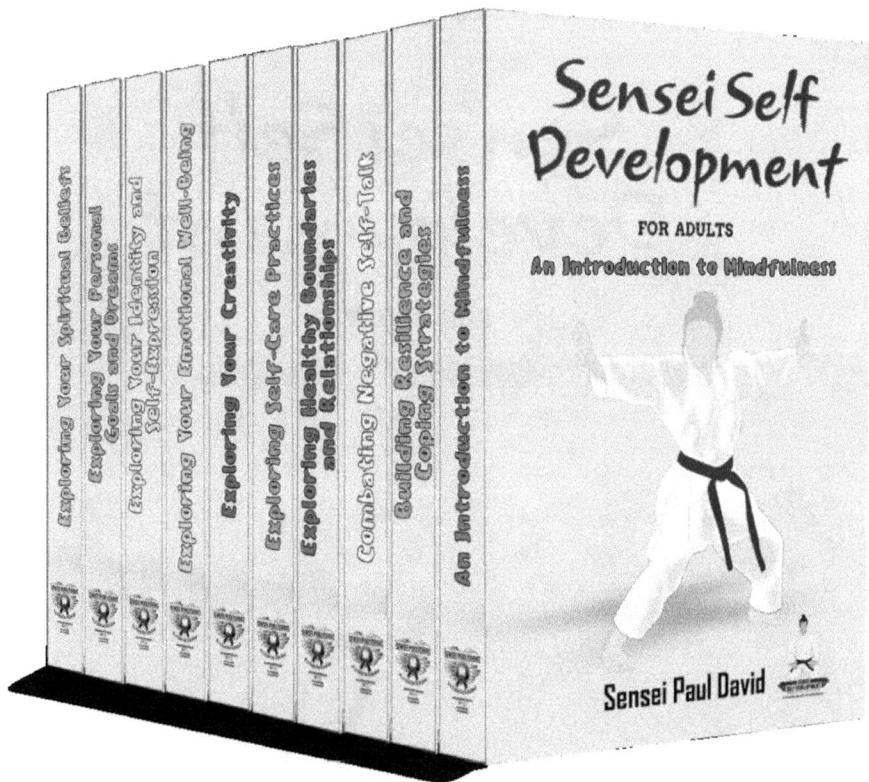

Exploring Your Spiritual Beliefs

Exploring Your Personal Goals and Dreams

Exploring Your Identity and Self-Expression

Exploring Your Emotional Well-Being

Exploring Your Creativity

Exploring Self-Care Practices

Exploring Healthy Boundaries and Relationships

Combatting Negative Self-Talk

Building Resilience and Coping Strategies

An Introduction to Mindfulness

Sensei Self Development

FOR ADULTS

An Introduction to Mindfulness

Sensei Paul David

Dedication

To those who courageously take action towards self-improvement - you are helping to evolve the world for generations to come.

- It's a great day to be alive!

If Found Please Contact:

_____

Reward If Found:

_____

MY
COMMITMENT

I, _____

commit   to   writing   This   Sensei   Self
Development Journal for at least 10 days in a
row, starting: _____

Writing this journal is valuable to me because:

_____

_____

_____

_____

_____

_____

If I finish a minimum of 10 consecutive days of
writing in this journal, I will reward myself by:

_____

_____

_____

_____

_____

_____

If I don't finish 10 days of writing this journal, I will promise to:

_____

_____

_____

_____

_____

I will do the following things to ensure that I write in my Sensei Self Development Journal every day:

_____

_____

_____

_____

_____

_____

Get/Share Your FREE All-Ages Mental Health eBook Now at

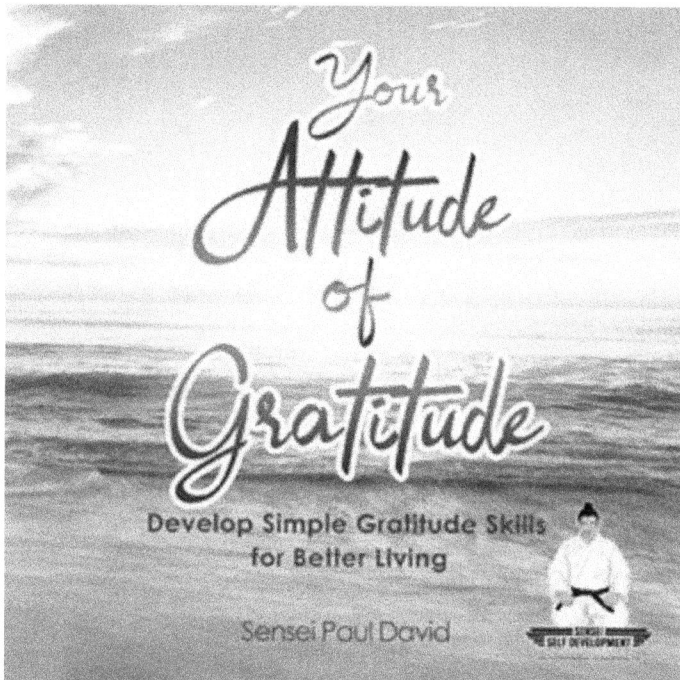

www.senseiselfdevelopment.com

Or CLICK HERE

Check Out Another Book In The SSD BOOK SERIES:

senseipublishing.com/SSD_SERIES

CLICK HERE

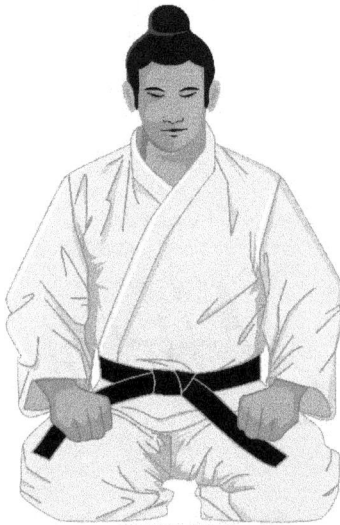

SENSEI
SELF DEVELOPMENT
BOOKS SERIES

senseiselfdevelopment.senseipublishing.com

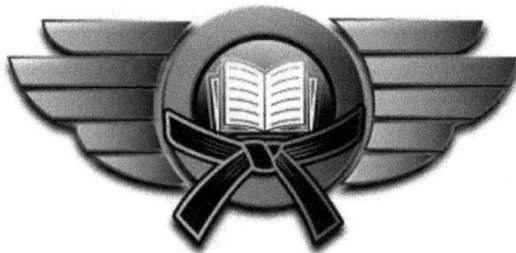

Join Our Publishing Journey!

If you would like to receive FUTURE FREE BOOKS and get to know us better, please click www.senseipublishing.com and join our newsletter by entering your email address in the pop-up box.

Follow Our Blog: senseipauldavid.ca

Follow/Like/Subscribe: Facebook, Instagram, YouTube: @senseipublishing

Scan the QR Code with your phone or tablet

to follow us on social media: Like / Subscribe / Follow

A Message From The Author:
Sensei Paul David

Dear Reader,

Welcome to the world of mental health journaling – a sacred space for self-reflection, growth, and healing. Within these pages, you hold the power to uplift your spirit, invigorate your mind, and nourish your goals.

In a world that often moves at blink-and-you'll-miss-it speed, it's crucial to make time for self-care and self-discovery.

Anxiety, stress, and emotional turbulence may have clouded your mind, making it difficult to find clarity and peace within. But fear not! Together, we will navigate the labyrinth of emotions, and experiences, helping to simplify the path to mental well-being.

This journal is not merely a bunch of blank pages awaiting your words. It is your compassionate companion, offering solace and understanding during your unique journey. Here, you are free to unburden yourself, celebrate small and large victories, and confront the challenges that may still linger.

Within the sheltered realm of these pages, there is no judgment, no expectation, and no pressure. Your unique experience and perspective hold immeasurable worth, and your voice deserves to be heard. Whether you choose to fill the lines with eloquence or simply scribble fragments of your thoughts, please remember each entry is a valuable contribution to your growth.

In this sacred space, you are challenged to take off the mask we so often wear in the outside world. It is here that you can be raw, vulnerable, and authentic – allowing your true self to be seen and embraced without reservation. By giving yourself permission to explore the depths of your emotions and confront the shadows that may lurk within, you will discover profound insights and find the healing you seek over time.

As you embark on this journaling journey, I encourage you to embrace the process itself rather than fixate solely on the outcome. Remember, it is not about reaching a certain destination or ticking off boxes on a list of accomplishments. Rather, it is about cultivating self-awareness, fostering self-compassion, and nurturing a sense of curiosity about the intricate workings of your intelligently beautiful mind.

In the quiet moments of reflection, let your pen become a bridge between your inner world and the possibilities that lie ahead. Create a sanctuary for your thoughts, fears, triumphs, and dreams. As you pour your heart onto these pages, allow your words to be a living testament to courage, resilience, and an unwavering commitment to your own well-being.

I am honored to be a part of your journey, and I believe in your ability to navigate the twists and turns with grace and resilience. Remember, you are not alone in this – countless others have walked similar paths, faced similar challenges, and emerged stronger and wiser on the other side. You have the power to reclaim all of your untapped joy, cultivate a positive mindset that serves you, and foster a deep sense of self-love and peaceful confident. – And it will take a worth effort and time.

So, open the first page of this journal with hope, curiosity, and an open heart and open mind. Embrace the transformative power of self-reflection, and allow it to guide you towards a life of greater fulfilment and peace. Each journaling session is an opportunity to not only connect with yourself but also to rekindle the light within that sometimes flickers but never extinguishes.

Remember, the pages you are about to fill are not just a record of your journey but also a testament to your strength, resilience, and indomitable spirit. Cherish this space, invest in yourself, and let your words be an ode to the magnificent journey of becoming whole.

With great respect for your decision to evolve,

Paul

MY CONVICTION

Please circle your answers below

I am DECIDING to be patient with myself and this PROCESS each time I journal toward my improved state of mental well-being

YES   NO

"The present moment is filled with joy and happiness. If you are attentive, you will see it."

Thich Nhat Hanh

Introduction

Self-doubt permeates various facets of our lives, influencing not only our personal self-perception but also how we interact with the broader world.

At its core, self-doubt is an internal dialogue, a questioning of one's abilities, decisions, and worth. It's a voice that whispers uncertainties and magnifies fears, often causing individuals to second-guess their actions and decisions.

This voice can be a fleeting thought before a significant choice or a persistent presence overshadowing daily life. It often arises at moments of vulnerability—when facing new challenges, stepping out of comfort zones, or when comparing oneself to others.

The prevalence of self-doubt is widespread, cutting across various demographics. Students, for instance, may grapple with it in academic settings, doubting their intelligence or the validity of their contributions. Artists and creatives might question their talent or the originality of their work, while professionals might feel it as 'imposter syndrome', doubting their qualifications or fearing exposure as a fraud.

The origins of self-doubt are multifaceted. It can stem from past experiences of failure or criticism, leading to a fear of repeating such scenarios.

Societal and cultural factors also play a significant role. In a world where success and perfection are often glorified, and failures are hidden, it's easy to feel inadequate or to believe that one is falling short of these high standards.

Moreover, the rise of social media, with its curated portrayals of success and happiness, adds another layer of comparison and self-scrutiny.

The impact of self-doubt extends beyond mere indecision or hesitation. It can lead to a cycle of negative thinking, affecting mental health and well-being. It might manifest as anxiety, stress, or a lack of motivation.

However, self-doubt isn't an insurmountable obstacle. It can be tamed. The journey begins with awareness. Awareness because problems like these, although great in stature, can blend in. They are like silent ghosts that pull on our strings without presenting themselves to us clearly. Their strength is in being hidden and they tend to melt under light of scrutiny.

In confronting self-doubt, introspection plays a vital role. This involves delving into the underlying causes of doubt - be it past experiences, fear of failure, or external pressures. By identifying these triggers, individuals can begin to challenge and dismantle the negative thought patterns that self-doubt breeds.

Another crucial aspect of overcoming self-doubt involves reshaping one's internal dialogue. This can be achieved through practices like mindfulness and Cognitive Behavioral techniques, which focus on recognizing and altering negative thought patterns.

Furthermore, embracing a learning mindset, where failures are seen as opportunities for growth, can significantly mitigate the impact of self-doubt. This shift in mindset involves understanding that perfection is an unrealistic goal and that mistakes are a natural part of the learning process. It encourages a focus on effort and improvement, rather than solely on outcomes.

Overcoming self-doubt is not about reaching a state where it no longer exists, but rather about developing the tools and resilience to manage it effectively. It's about building a relationship with doubt where it serves as a checkpoint, prompting reflection and caution, rather than a roadblock.

Ultimately, the journey through self-doubt is a path towards greater self-assurance and fulfillment. It's a process of learning to trust one's abilities and to understand that doubt, while a natural part of the human experience, doesn't define one's capabilities or worth.

The Impact of Self-Doubt

Self-doubt is a natural cognitive process where you question your abilities and decisions. When you're about to do something new or challenging, your brain starts to assess the risks and your capability to handle them. This questioning can be healthy, as it helps in evaluating decisions carefully. But when it tips over into persistent self-questioning, it can lead to a significant drop in confidence.

This decline in confidence is not just a feeling. It's backed by neuroscience. When you doubt yourself, your brain can actually limit the neural pathways that help in decision-making and problem-solving. It's similar to how a computer runs slower when too many applications are open. Your brain, bogged down by self-doubt, struggles to operate efficiently.

The impact of this on decision-making is profound. Faced with choices, your brain, influenced by self-doubt, tends to overanalyze, leading to decision paralysis. It's not merely indecision; it's your brain's way of trying to avoid potential mistakes, a protective mechanism that sometimes goes into overdrive.

In terms of relationships, self-doubt activates the brain's social monitoring systems. You become more attuned to reactions and feedback from others, interpreting them in the context of your doubts. This heightened sensitivity can lead to misinterpretations, where you might perceive disappointment or disapproval even when none exists.

In the workplace, self-doubt triggers the brain's stress responses. This can manifest as impostor syndrome, where despite evidence of your competencies, your brain is convinced that you're not as capable as others perceive you to be. This internal conflict can lead to chronic stress, affecting both mental and physical health.

Creativity and self-doubt have a complex relationship. Creative endeavors require risk-taking and embracing the unknown – things that self-doubt often stifles. When you doubt your creative abilities, it can limit your brain's ability to think outside the box, reducing the flow of creative ideas.

But self-doubt isn't all bad. In moderation, it can be a useful cognitive tool. It encourages the brain to double-check and refine thoughts and decisions, acting as a balance to overconfidence. The key is in managing self-doubt so it doesn't dominate your thought processes. Mindfulness and cognitive-behavioral strategies can be effective in keeping self-doubt in check, ensuring it doesn't hinder your potential.

All in all, Self-doubt is a natural, albeit sometimes overactive, brain function. It's a common human experience, and learning to navigate it is a part of personal growth. Remember, the goal isn't to eliminate self-doubt entirely but to manage it in a way that it becomes a constructive part of your decision-making process.

How to Overcome Self-Doubt

Behavioural Experiments

Behavioral experiments involve testing the beliefs that fuel our insecurities in real-world scenarios, but in a manageable and controlled way. This method allows us to gather evidence about our thoughts and beliefs, helping us see them in a new light.

Let's say you've always doubted your ability to make new friends. You think, "If I go to that social event, I won't connect with anyone." Here's where a behavioral experiment comes in. You decide to attend the event with the intention of simply observing what happens. Maybe you set a small, achievable goal like initiating a conversation with just one person. The experiment is not about proving your doubt right or wrong but about exploring what actually happens.

Or consider public speaking, a common source of anxiety and self-doubt. You're tasked with giving a presentation and your mind buzzes with thoughts like, "I'll mess up and everyone will think less of me." To experiment, you might focus on just one aspect of the task – maybe maintaining eye contact or keeping a steady pace. Afterwards, you reflect on the experience. Did the audience react as negatively as you expected? Often, you'll find the reality is far less daunting than your predictions.

Another example could be related to your skills at work. Perhaps you doubt your competence in a certain area. You might test this by volunteering for a project that requires these skills, but in a low-stakes setting.

This approach allows you to gather real evidence about your abilities, rather than relying on unfounded self-doubt.

The beauty of these experiments lies in their simplicity and their power to reveal new perspectives. Each time you conduct one, you gather a little more evidence that challenges your self-doubt. You learn that outcomes are rarely as dire as your doubts suggest, and that you're more capable than you give yourself credit for.

It's important to approach these experiments with kindness and patience towards yourself. They are not about pushing yourself into uncomfortable situations without support or care. Instead, think of them as opportunities for growth, understanding, and self-compassion. As you continue on this path, you'll likely find that the weight of self-doubt becomes lighter, and the confidence in your steps grows stronger.

Channel Your Alter Ego

Before becoming famous as Dice, Andrew Clay Silverstein was a young boy growing up in Brooklyn, New York. He had a close-knit family and loved performing, often impersonating celebrities like John Travolta and Jerry Lewis.

John Travolta's character Danny Zuko in "Grease" inspired Clay, leading him to adopt Zuko's style, including the iconic leather jacket and slicked-back hair.

Clay worked hard in various fields, but comedy was his true passion. With the help of fellow comedian Michael Blinder, his character "Dice" was born in the early 1980s, a tough-talking Italian-American. This transformation wasn't just on stage; it started to blur the lines between his persona and real life.

Living as Dice made Clay feel more alive and in control, which led to greater confidence. This concept of adopting an alter ego can help boost confidence, but it has its risks. In Clay's case, he became confident but also adopted negative traits from Dice, like sexism and irrational behavior.

When creating an alter ego, it's essential to be mindful of the traits you emulate and avoid extremes. Drawing inspiration from bold, confident personalities can help, but be aware of potential pitfalls.

Be Hyper Honest

On the surface, it might be difficult to see how honesty might correlate to self-doubt. But it does. Have you ever been in a situation where you lied or skewed the truth because you were embarrassed. It could be asking your dad to park your car farther from your high school, or not speaking for a piece of music you like as your friend trashed it. Or it could be a straight up lie, like you did not fart when you did.

But imagine if you spoke up. And said to your friends "You guys don't know anything about music. I freaking love this song". And you admitted, with maybe a devilish smile on your face, that you were the one who let one out. Maybe you drove your trashy car with confidence and did not try to hide it.

Of course, this does not mean you have to be shameless. You can still hold your tongue or say something in a nice way because it is an appropriate way to communicate. But altering your speech because you are embarrassed or afraid to be judged for your way of life or opinions is a big NO-NO.

When you are hyper honest and tell people like it is without any care, you feel empowered. Standing up for your taste is empowering. Not shying away from your identity, your beliefs, the way your family does things makes you feel more confident and less doubtful about yourself. Try it. And you will see.

Try Cognitive Reframing

Cognitive reframing is a technique used to change the way you think about a situation or problem in order to reduce negative emotions and improve your outlook. It involves looking at things from a different perspective or "reframing" them in a more positive or constructive light.

For example, Imagine you're about to give a presentation at work, and self-doubt starts creeping in. Instead of thinking, "I'm going to mess this up; I'm terrible at presenting," try reframing it as, "I've prepared for this presentation, and I know my material well. I might feel nervous, but that's normal. It's a chance to showcase my knowledge and improve my public speaking skills." This change in mindset can help you manage self-doubt and perform better in real-life situations.

Here's how you can use cognitive reframing:

1. The first step is to catch yourself when you're thinking negatively. It might be thoughts like "I can't do this" or "I'm not good enough." Recognize these thoughts as they happen.

2. Once you identify a negative thought, ask yourself, is this really true? Often, these thoughts are based on fear, not reality. Challenge their validity. For instance, if you think, "I always fail," remind yourself of the times you've succeeded.

3. This is where you change the narrative. Turn "I can't do this" into "I can do this with some effort and learning." It's not about ignoring your limits, but about seeing your potential and growth. You don't have to lie to yourself. Being honest is enough.

4. Like any skill, cognitive reframing takes practice. The more you do it, the more natural it becomes. Over time, you'll find that positive thoughts start to grow more naturally in your mind-garden, keeping the weeds of self-doubt at bay.

Remember, it's okay if it feels a bit forced at first. With time and practice, cognitive reframing can become a natural part of your thought process, helping you to overcome self-doubt and view challenges in a more positive light.

Try things that make you uncomfortable

To deal with self-doubt, it's important to try new things, even if they make you uncomfortable. Start by understanding that doing things outside your comfort zone is hard, but it helps you grow. Try doing things you don't normally do, like talking to new people if you're shy, trying different foods if you always eat the same thing, or taking on new responsibilities at work or addressing problems in your personal life. This can boost your confidence and make you feel better about yourself.

Doing these things will tell your mind that you can do them and it does not have to be worried. So it will calm down. It will start trusting your judgement. And start accepting that this is how things go. You will always have a certain level of doubt. That's for sure. But it will be way less. And as you achieve more little trophies, they will keep the self doubt at bay so that it does not consume you into fear and ultimately inaction.

The emphasis here is on gradual progression rather than abrupt, overwhelming changes. For instance, if you're shy, you might start by striking up a brief conversation with a colleague. If you're apprehensive about new culinary experiences, you could begin by trying a dish that includes one unfamiliar ingredient. In professional or personal settings, taking on tasks that you would usually avoid can help you build resilience and confidence.

By continuously pushing your boundaries in these small but significant ways, you incrementally expand your comfort zone. Over time, what once felt daunting becomes less intimidating, and you start to develop a sense of ease in a variety of situations. This expanded comfort zone is essential for personal development, as it equips you with the confidence and adaptability needed to navigate diverse and challenging scenarios with less self-doubt and more assurance.

Defy Imposter syndrome

Impostor syndrome is a psychological pattern where individuals doubt their accomplishments, often feeling like they're not as competent as others perceive them to be. Despite evident success, they might fear being exposed as a "fraud." This syndrome is common and can affect anyone, regardless of their skill level or expertise.

To counter impostor syndrome, a proactive approach is maintaining a record of your achievements. This involves setting up a dedicated notebook or a digital file where you regularly jot down your successes. These can be small wins, like successfully navigating a challenging situation, or significant triumphs, such as completing a major project or acquiring a new skill.

By documenting these accomplishments, you create a tangible reminder of your capabilities, which helps in shifting your focus from self-doubt to self-recognition. Over time, this habit not only bolsters your confidence but also provides a concrete counter-narrative to the feelings of being an impostor, reminding you of the real and valuable contributions you've made.

Understanding the Role of Time

When you're just starting out with a new skill, whether it's driving, cooking, or playing an instrument, it's natural that your first attempts won't be flawless. This is a normal part of the learning process. Expecting to excel immediately is not only unrealistic but also sets you up for unnecessary self-doubt.

It's important to note that even when you become more adept at a skill, doubts can still arise, but they often take on a different form. Take the example of a chef. A novice chef might doubt their basic abilities in the kitchen, questioning whether they can cook edible meals. However, an experienced chef's doubts are less about their fundamental skills and more about the nuances and uncertainties inherent in cooking, like experimenting with new recipes or ingredients. The nature of their doubt has evolved from questioning their basic ability to exploring the boundaries of their expertise.

Consider a new chef comparing their sushi to that made by a renowned sushi master. The new chef might feel disheartened, thinking their sushi is inadequate. But if they remind themselves that the sushi master likely has years, if not decades, of experience, it can put things into perspective. The new chef's sushi, after one year of practice, is exactly where it should be. Their current skill level is appropriate for their experience, and with time and practice, they can aspire to reach higher levels of mastery.

The key is to always remember the role of time. Skills and expertise are not acquired overnight. They are the result of consistent effort, practice, and, most importantly, time. Forgetting this – the invisible aspect of time that goes into honing a skill – is what often leads to self-doubt. By acknowledging and respecting the time required, we can set more realistic expectations for ourselves and reduce unnecessary doubts about our abilities.

Self-compassion for Overcoming Self-Doubt

Self-compassion is like being your own best friend, especially when facing self-doubt. It's about treating yourself with the same kindness and understanding you'd offer to someone you care about. Here's how you can practice self-compassion:

1. Recognizing Common Humanity: Imagine you're sitting with a friend who's sharing their doubts and mistakes. You'd likely say, "Hey, we all go through this." That's the essence of recognizing our common humanity. When you feel self-doubt creeping in, remind yourself that you're not alone. Everyone has these moments, and it's a normal part of being human.

2. Kind Self-Talk: Think of how you talk to a loved one when they're down. Now, try turning that kindness inward. Instead of beating yourself up with thoughts like, "I can't do

anything right," try a gentler approach: "I'm doing my best, and that's okay." It's about being your own supportive friend.

3. Mindfulness: This is like sitting by a river and watching your thoughts and feelings flow by. You notice them, you acknowledge them, but you don't jump in and let them sweep you away. If you're feeling overwhelmed, take a moment to breathe and say to yourself, "It's okay to feel this way. It's a part of life."

4. Self-Care Practices: It could be as simple as enjoying a quiet cup of tea, reading a book, or taking a walk in nature. It all depends on what you feel soothing and self assuring. These moments of care add up, helping you to feel grounded and valued.

5. Forgive Yourself: Forgiveness is like a warm, comforting light on a cold day. We all make mistakes, and that's how we learn and grow. When something doesn't go as planned, wrap

yourself in understanding and say, "It's alright. I'm still learning."

Journaling

When you're feeling doubtful, grab a notebook and let your thoughts flow onto the page. There's something magical about the act of writing—it helps to untangle thoughts, providing clarity and insight.

Start by describing what you're feeling. Are you doubting your abilities at work? Are you questioning your decisions? Write it all down, as if you're telling a story. This process in itself can be incredibly freeing. It's like lifting a weight off your shoulders and placing it on the paper.

Then, you can start to explore these feelings. Ask yourself why you feel this way. Often, we discover that our self-doubt is rooted in deeper fears or past experiences. Writing this down can help you understand the source of your doubts, making them less intimidating.

As you continue to write, try to shift your perspective. If you've written down a negative thought, see if you can challenge it. For instance, if you've written, "I always mess things up," consider moments where you've succeeded. Write about these successes, however small they may be. This act of reflection can slowly start to change the narrative in your head.

You can also use journaling to visualize and plan. Write about where you want to be, how you want to feel. Set small, achievable goals for yourself and jot down steps on how you can reach them. This not only provides a sense of direction but also a path that you can look back on to see how far you've come.

Remember, your journal is a safe space. It's a place of non-judgment. Whether you write a few lines or pages, what matters is that you're taking the time to connect with and understand yourself. Over time, you might find that this practice becomes a comforting ritual, a way to soothe and overcome the waves of self-doubt, turning them into a sea of self-awareness and confidence.

Before We Get Started…

Remember, mindfulness journaling is a personal practice, and these questions are meant to guide and inspire you. Feel free to adapt and modify them to suit your needs and preferences. Explore, reflect, and embrace the opportunity to deepen your self-awareness and cultivate a sense of inner peace.

Date ___ / ___ / ___ : S   M   T   W   Th   F   S

I feel:
(please circle)

because   because   because   because   because
_____   _____   _____   _____   _____
_____   _____   _____   _____   _____

Today I Am Grateful For

1. _____
2. _____
3. _____

What could help transform today into a remarkable day?

Reflective Writing

How do you recognize when you are experiencing self-doubt?

_____

_____

_____

_____

_____

_____

_____

What is one effective way to overcome self-doubt?

A) Practice positive self-talk

B) Isolate oneself from others

C) Avoid seeking help from others

D) Compare oneself to others

All Are Correct - Choose The Response You Feel Is Most Important To Remember

Date ___ / ___ / ___ : S M T W Th F S

I feel:
(please circle)

because   because   because   because   because
_____   _____   _____   _____   _____
_____

Today I Am Grateful For

1. _____
2. _____
3. _____

What could help transform today into a remarkable day?

Reflective Writing

What strategies have you used to overcome self-doubt?

_____

_____

_____

_____

_____

_____

_____

What is the main difference between self-doubt and low self-esteem?

A) Self-doubt is temporary while low self-esteem is long-lasting

B) Self-doubt is internal while low self-esteem is external

C) Self-doubt has a positive impact while low self-esteem has a negative impact

D) Self-doubt is situational while low self-esteem is a consistent belief

All Are Correct - Choose The Response You Feel Is Most Important To Remember

Date ___ / ___ / ___ : S M T W Th F S

I feel:
(please circle)

because   because   because   because   because
_____   _____   _____   _____   _____
_____   _____   _____   _____   _____

Today I Am Grateful For

1. _____
2. _____
3. _____

What could help transform today into a remarkable day?

Reflective Writing

How do you challenge negative thoughts that lead
to self-doubt and low self-esteem?

_____

_____

_____

_____

_____

_____

_____

Which statement is true about self-doubt and self-esteem?

A) They can both arise from external influences

B) They are both permanent mindsets

C) They have no impact on one's actions

D) They are unrelated to one's well-being

All Are Correct - Choose The Response You Feel Is Most Important To Remember

Date ___ / ___ / ___ : S M T W Th F S

I feel: (please circle)

because | because | because | because | because
_____ | _____ | _____ | _____ | _____
_____ | _____ | _____ | _____ | _____

Today I Am Grateful For

1. _____
2. _____
3. _____

What could help transform today into a remarkable day?

Reflective Writing

What techniques have you used to build self-confidence?

_____

_____

_____

_____

_____

_____

_____

How can self-doubt affect an individual's daily life?

A) It can lead to increased productivity
B) It can cause feelings of incompetence
C) It can improve decision-making abilities
D) It can foster healthy relationships with others

All Are Correct - Choose The Response You Feel Is Most Important To Remember

Date ___ / ___ / ___ : S M T W Th F S

I feel:
(please circle)

because because because because because
_____ _____ _____ _____ _____
_____ _____ _____ _____ _____

Today I Am Grateful For

1. _____
2. _____
3. _____

What could help transform today into a remarkable day?

Reflective Writing

What positive self-talk do you use to boost your self-esteem?

_____

_____

_____

_____

_____

_____

_____

What is one effective way to improve self-esteem?

A) Criticize oneself regularly

B) Surround oneself with negative influences

C) Acknowledge and build upon one's strengths

D) Focus on one's weaknesses and flaws

All Are Correct - Choose The Response You Feel Is Most Important To Remember

Date ___ / ___ / ___ : S   M   T   W   Th   F   S

I feel:
(please circle)

because _____ because _____ because _____ because _____ because _____
_____ _____ _____ _____ _____

Today I Am Grateful For

1. _____
2. _____
3. _____

What could help transform today into a remarkable day?

Reflective Writing

How do you recognize and challenge the limiting beliefs that lead to self-doubt?

_____

_____

_____

_____

_____

_____

_____

How can seeking validation from others contribute to self-doubt?

A) It can reinforce negative thoughts and beliefs

B) It can lead to increased confidence

C) It can improve one's self-awareness

D) It can help determine one's own worth

All Are Correct - Choose The Response You Feel Is Most Important To Remember

Date ___ / ___ / ___: S   M   T   W   Th   F   S

I feel:
(please circle)

because   because   because   because   because
_____   _____   _____   _____   _____
_____

Today I Am Grateful For

1. _____
2. _____
3. _____

What could help transform today into a remarkable day?

Reflective Writing

How do you stay motivated to keep working on improving your self-esteem?

_____

_____

_____

_____

_____

_____

_____

What is one common cause of low self-esteem?

A) Negative self-talk
B) Positive feedback from others
C) Accomplishing goals
D) Social media validation

All Are Correct - Choose The Response You Feel Is Most Important
To Remember

Date ___ / ___ / ___: S M T W Th F S

I feel:
(please circle)

because because because because because
_____ _____ _____ _____ _____
_____ _____ _____ _____ _____

Today I Am Grateful For

1. _____
2. _____
3. _____

What could help transform today into a remarkable day?

Reflective Writing

How do you recognize and respond to negative influences that contribute to self-doubt?

_____

_____

_____

_____

_____

_____

_____

_____

How can setting realistic goals help overcome self-doubt and low self-esteem?

A) It can prevent one from experiencing failure

B) It can provide a sense of purpose and achievement

C) It can increase self-criticism and doubt

D) It can make one feel inadequate and incapable

All Are Correct - Choose The Response You Feel Is Most Important To Remember

Date ___ / ___ / ___ : S   M   T   W   Th   F   S

I feel:
(please circle)

because   because   because   because   because
_____   _____   _____   _____   _____
_____   _____   _____   _____   _____

Today I Am Grateful For

1. _____
2. _____
3. _____

What could help transform today into a remarkable day?

Reflective Writing

How do you practice self-care to combat self-doubt and low self-esteem?

_____

_____

_____

_____

_____

_____

_____

How can comparing oneself to others negatively impact self-esteem?

A) It can motivate one to work harder and achieve more
B) It can lead to feelings of inadequacy and self-doubt
C) It can improve one's self-confidence and self-worth
D) It can help identify areas for self-improvement

All Are Correct - Choose The Response You Feel Is Most Important To Remember

Date ___ / ___ / ___ : S M T W Th F S

I feel:
(please circle)

because because because because because

_____ _____ _____ _____ _____

_____ _____ _____ _____ _____

Today I Am Grateful For

1. _____

2. _____

3. _____

What could help transform today into a remarkable day?

Reflective Writing

How do you set realistic goals to help build self-confidence?

_____

_____

_____

_____

_____

_____

_____

What is one effective way to silence negative self-talk?

A) Share one's doubts and insecurities with others

B) Write down and challenge negative thoughts

C) Ignore and suppress negative thoughts

D) Surround oneself with people who criticize and put one down

All Are Correct - Choose The Response You Feel Is Most Important To Remember

Date ___ / ___ / ___ : S M T W Th F S

I feel:
(please circle)

because   because   because   because   because
_____   _____   _____   _____   _____
_____   _____   _____   _____   _____

Today I Am Grateful For

1. _____
2. _____
3. _____

What could help transform today into a remarkable day?

Reflective Writing

What techniques do you use to manage stress
that can contribute to self-doubt?

_____

_____

_____

_____

_____

_____

_____

How can self-care practices improve self-esteem and reduce self-doubt?

A) They can increase one's dependence on others

B) They can help one become more self-critical

C) They can promote self-love and self-acceptance

D) They can create a sense of competition and inadequacy

All Are Correct - Choose The Response You Feel Is Most Important To Remember

Date ___ / ___ / ___ : S M T W Th F S

I feel:
(please circle)

because _____ because _____ because _____ because _____ because _____
_____ _____ _____ _____ _____

Today I Am Grateful For

1. _____
2. _____
3. _____

What could help transform today into a remarkable day?

Reflective Writing
How do you celebrate your successes and build self-belief?

_____

_____

_____

_____

_____

_____

_____

What is one way to overcome the fear of failure and self-doubt?

A) Avoid taking any risks or trying new things
B) Set unrealistic and unattainable goals
C) Accept and learn from failures
D) Constantly seek approval and validation from others

All Are Correct - Choose The Response You Feel Is Most Important To Remember

Date ___ / ___ / ___: S M T W Th F S

I feel: (please circle)

because _____ because _____ because _____ because _____ because _____

Today I Am Grateful For

1. _____
2. _____
3. _____

What could help transform today into a remarkable day?

Reflective Writing
How do you recognize and challenge the self-defeating behaviors that contribute to self-doubt?

_____

_____

_____

_____

_____

_____

_____

How can self-compassion help improve self-esteem?

A) It can lead to feelings of selfishness and narcissism

B) It can decrease feelings of guilt and shame

C) It can increase feelings of inadequacy and incompetence

D) It can improve one's relationships with others

All Are Correct - Choose The Response You Feel Is Most Important To Remember

Date ___ / ___ / ___ : S   M   T   W   Th   F   S

I feel:
(please circle)

because   because   because   because   because

_____   _____   _____   _____   _____

_____   _____   _____   _____   _____

Today I Am Grateful For

1. _____
2. _____
3. _____

What could help transform today into a remarkable day?

Reflective Writing

How do you practice positive self-affirmation to build self-esteem?

_____

_____

_____

_____

_____

_____

_____

_____

What is the first step in overcoming self-doubt and building self-esteem?

A) Seeking validation from others
B) Setting impossible goals
C) Identifying and challenging negative thoughts
D) Comparing oneself to others

All Are Correct - Choose The Response You Feel Is Most Important To Remember

Date ___ / ___ / ___ : S M T W Th F S

I feel:
(please circle)

because   because   because   because   because

_____   _____   _____   _____   _____

_____   _____   _____   _____   _____

Today I Am Grateful For

1. _____

2. _____

3. _____

What could help transform today into a remarkable day?

Reflective Writing

How do you recognize and combat feelings of fear and
insecurity that lead to self-doubt?

_____

_____

_____

_____

_____

_____

_____

How can a supportive and positive social circle positively impact self-esteem?

A) It can make one feel undeserving of support and love

B) It can provide a sense of belonging and acceptance

C) It can increase feelings of isolation and inadequacy

D) It can lead to unhealthy competition and self-comparison

All Are Correct - Choose The Response You Feel Is Most Important To Remember

As we reach the final pages of this journey through "Positive Mindset," I want to extend my heartfelt thanks to you. Your commitment to exploring positivity and its transformative power is not only commendable but a testament to your desire for personal growth and a richer, more fulfilling life experience.

Remember, the journey towards a positive mindset is ongoing and ever-evolving. Each day presents new opportunities to apply these principles, to learn, and to grow. I encourage you to revisit these pages whenever you need a reminder of your incredible potential to foster positivity and resilience in the face of life's challenges.

As we part ways, I leave you with a quote that has been a guiding star in my journey: "The greatest discovery of any generation is that a human can alter his life by altering his attitude."

– William James.

Thank you for allowing me to be a part of your journey. May your path be filled with light, hope, and endless possibilities. Farewell, and may you carry the spirit of positivity with you, today and always.

With gratitude and best wishes,

Sensei Paul David

Reflective Writing

The End

As you close the pages of this mindfulness journal, remember that each word you've written is a step on your journey towards self-awareness and inner peace. Embrace the moments of clarity, the revelations, and even the uncertainties you've encountered along the way. Let this journal be a testament to your growth and a reminder that every day offers a new opportunity to be present, to observe, and to appreciate the simple wonders of life. Carry these lessons forward, and may your path be filled with mindful moments and serene reflections. Until we meet again in these pages, be gentle with yourself and stay anchored in the now.

Mindfulness isn't difficult, we just need to remember to do it.

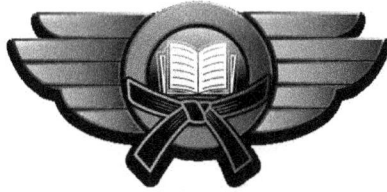

Thank You!

If you found this book helpful, I would be grateful if you would **post an honest review on Amazon** so this book can reach other supportive readers like you!

All you need to do is digitally flip to the back and leave your review. Or visit amazon.com/author/senseipauldavid click the correct book cover and click on the blue link next to the yellow stars that say, "customer reviews."

As always...
It's a great day to be alive!

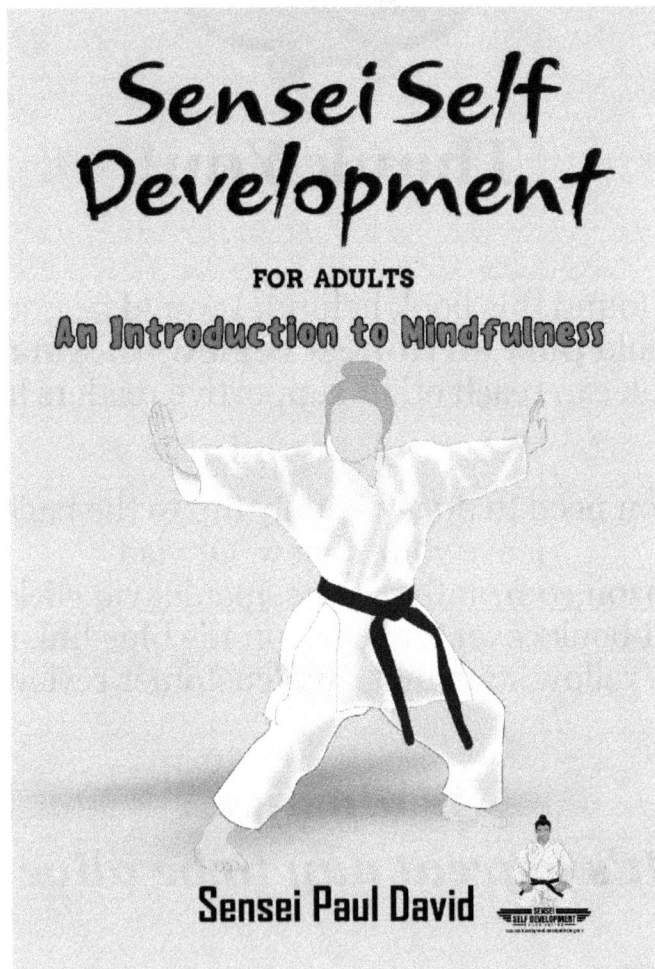

Sensei Self Development

FOR ADULTS

An Introduction to Mindfulness

Sensei Paul David

Check Out The SSD Chronicles
Series CLICK HERE

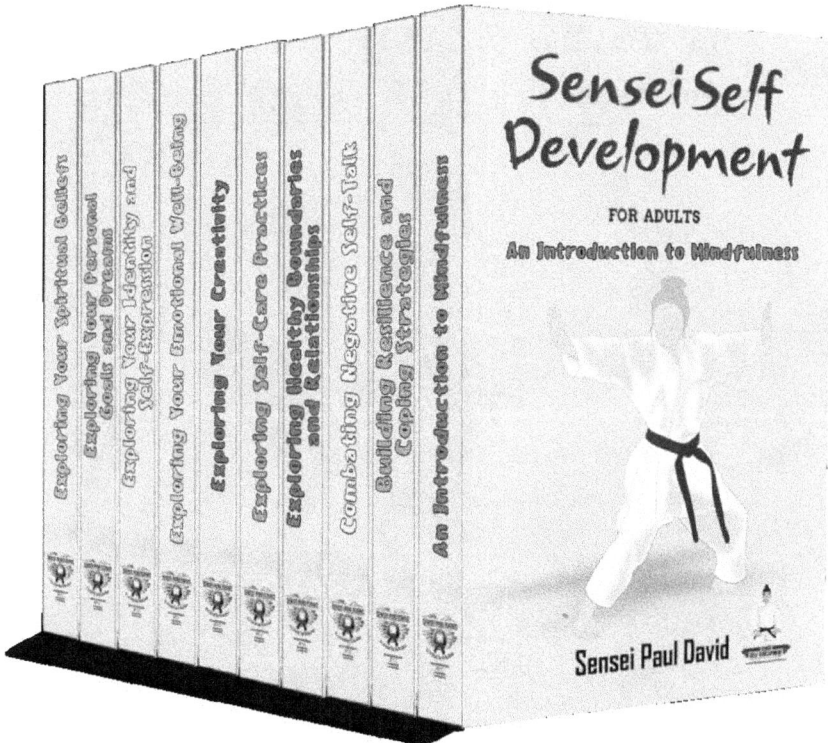

Get/Share Your FREE All-Ages Mental Health eBook Now at

www.senseiselfdevelopment.com

Or CLICK HERE

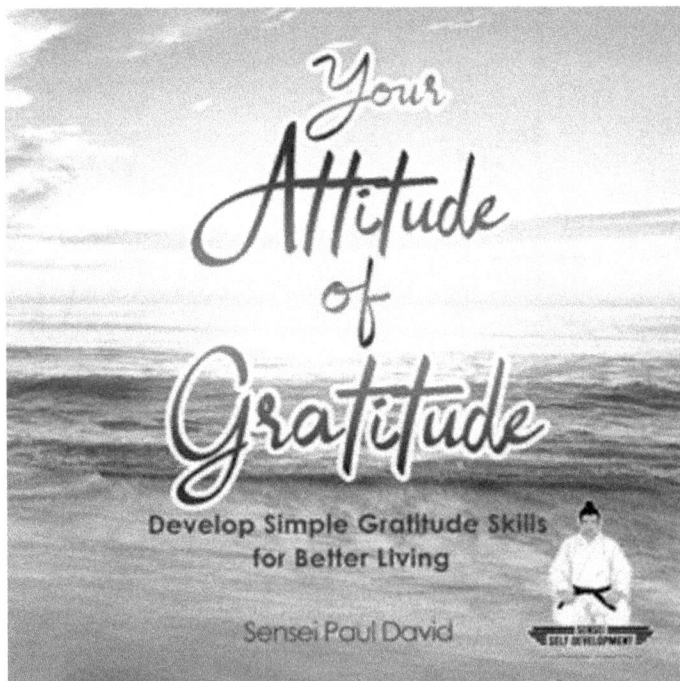

senseiselfdevelopment.com

Click Another Book In The SSD BOOK SERIES:

senseipublishing.com/SSD_SERIES

CLICK HERE

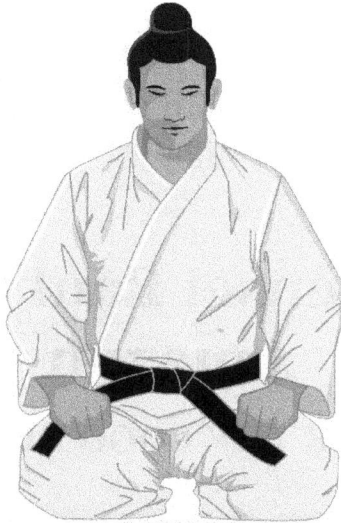

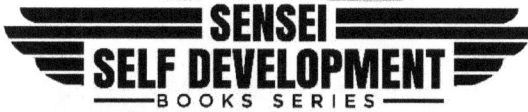

senseiselfdevelopment.senseipublishing.com

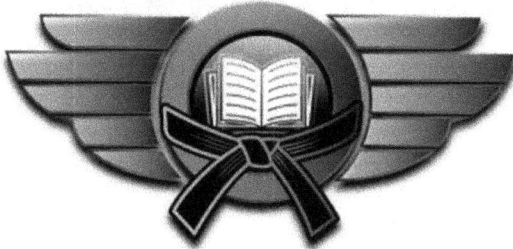

Join Our Publishing Journey!

If you would like to receive FREE BOOKS, please visit **www.senseipublishing.com**. Join our newsletter by entering your email address in the pop-up box

Follow Sensei Paul David on Amazon

CLICK THE LOGO BELOW

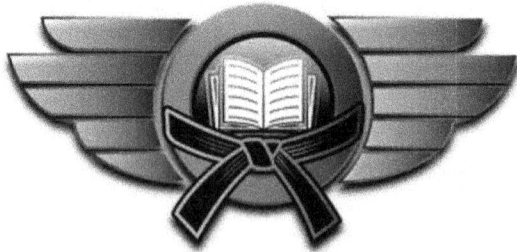

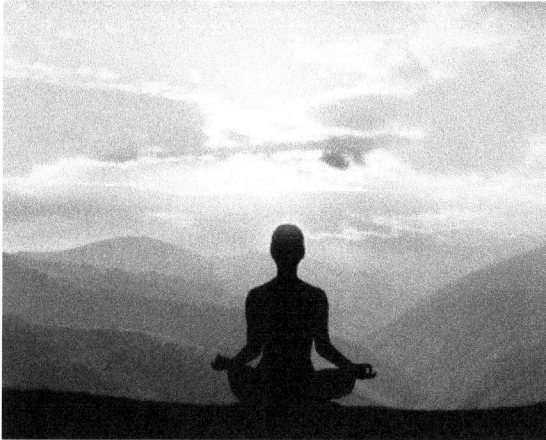

FREE BONUS!!!
Experience Over 25 FREE Engaging Guided Meditations!

Prized Skills & Practices for Adults & Kids. Help Restore Deep-Sleep, Lower Stress, Improve Posture, Navigate Uncertainty & More.

Download the Free Insight Timer App and click the link below:
http://insig.ht/sensei_paul

About Sensei Publishing

Sensei Publishing commits itself to helping people of all ages transform into better versions of themselves by providing high-quality and research-based self-development books with an emphasis on mental health and guided meditations. Sensei Publishing offers well-written e-books, audiobooks, paperbacks and online courses that simplify complicated but practical topics in line with its mission to inspire people towards positive transformation.

It's a great day to be alive!

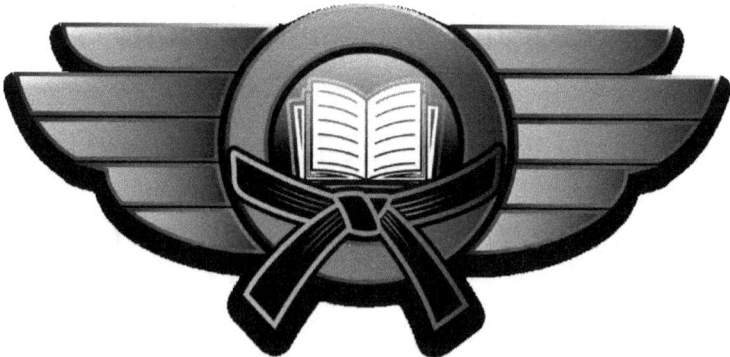

About the Author

I create simple & transformative eBooks & Guided Meditations for Adults & Children proven to help navigate uncertainty, solve niche problems & bring families closer together.

I'm a former finance project manager, private pilot, jiu-jitsu instructor, musician & former University of Toronto Fitness Trainer. I prefer a science-based approach to focus on these & other areas in my life to stay humble & hungry to evolve. I hope you enjoy my work and I'd love to hear your feedback.

- It's a great day to be alive!

Sensei Paul David

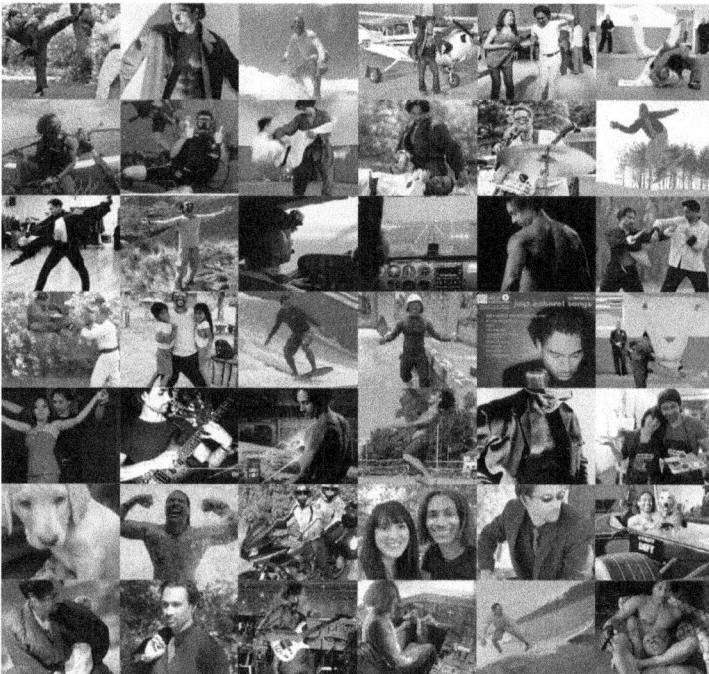

Scan & Follow/Like/Subscribe: Facebook, Instagram,
YouTube: @senseipublishing

Scan using your phone/iPad camera for Social Media
Visit us at www.senseipublishing.com and sign up for our
newsletter to learn more about our exciting books and to
experience our FREE Guided Meditations for Kids & Adults.